Alexander Wellington

Sweet Success

Empowering
Children
with Type 1
Diabetes

Steps to Success

1. Understanding Type 1 Diabetes
  - Overview of type 1 diabetes
  - Causes and symptoms
  - Diagnosis and initial steps

2. The Importance of Diabetes Management
  - Long-term effects of unmanaged diabetes
  - Benefits of proactive management
  - Setting goals for effective management

3. Building a Supportive Environment
  - Family support and involvement
  - School support and education
  - Community resources and support groups

4. Blood Glucose Monitoring
  - Importance of regular monitoring
  - Techniques for blood glucose testing
  - Interpreting blood glucose results

5. Insulin Therapy
  - Types of insulin and their action profiles
  - Insulin administration methods
  - Insulin dosage calculation and adjustments

6. Nutrition and Meal Planning

- Understanding carbohydrates, proteins, and fats
- Meal planning strategies for balanced nutrition
- Managing blood sugar levels through diet

Chart: Common Foods and their Nutrition Facts

7. Physical Activity and Diabetes

- Benefits of exercise for diabetes management
- Exercise guidelines and precautions
- Balancing insulin, food, and exercise

8. Managing Diabetes at School

- Communicating with school staff about diabetes
- Creating a diabetes management plan for school
- Addressing challenges and advocating for your child's needs

9. Handling Emotional and Social Challenges

- Coping with the emotional impact of diabetes
- Dealing with peer pressure and stigma
- Building resilience and self-esteem

10. Emergencies and Complications

- Recognizing and managing hypoglycemia
- Dealing with hyperglycemia and diabetic ketoacidosis
- Preventing and managing diabetes-related complications

11. Technology and Diabetes Management
- Continuous glucose monitoring (CGM) systems
- Insulin pumps and automated insulin delivery systems
- Integrating technology into daily diabetes care

12. Transitioning to Independence
- Teaching self-care skills to children
- Gradual transition to independent diabetes management
- Supporting adolescents in managing their diabetes responsibly

13. Living a Full Life with Diabetes
- Pursuing hobbies and interests
- Traveling with diabetes
- Balancing diabetes management with everyday life

14. Celebrating Successes and Milestones
- Recognizing achievements in diabetes management
- Setting and reaching milestones
- Fostering a positive outlook on living with diabetes

15. Looking Towards the Future
- Advances in diabetes research and treatment
- Hope for a cure
- Empowering children and families to thrive despite diabetes
- Cultivating Resilience
- Inspiring Change

Prologue

In the quiet hours before dawn, a child's world changed forever. It was in the hushed moments of a hospital room, amid beeping monitors and whispered consultations, that a family first confronted the unwelcome intruder—Diabetes.

For them, and for countless families around the world, this diagnosis marked the beginning of an uncharted journey, illuminated by moments of courage, resilience, and unwavering determination.

In the pages that follow, we embark on a voyage—not only through the intricacies of managing a chronic condition but also through the depths of the human spirit. It's a journey of love, of setbacks and triumphs, bound by the unwavering resolve to empower our children, to equip them with the tools they need to thrive despite the odds.

As we navigate the twists and turns of this path, we discover that while diabetes may alter the landscape of our lives, it does not define us. It is but a chapter in the story— filled with uncertainty, yes, but also with hope, with strength, and with the unshakeable belief that together, we can conquer even the most formidable of challenges.

So, dear reader, as you turn the page and step into the world of "Sweet Success: Empowering Children with Type 1 Diabetes," remember this: within these pages lie not just words, but the collective wisdom, the shared experiences, and the unwavering spirit of a community united in its quest for hope, for resilience, and for sweet success.

Chapter 1

Type 1 Diabetes, often referred to as juvenile diabetes, is a chronic autoimmune condition characterized by the body's inability to produce insulin, the hormone responsible for regulating blood sugar levels. Unlike Type 2 Diabetes, which is commonly associated with lifestyle factors like obesity and physical inactivity, Type 1 Diabetes typically manifests in childhood or adolescence and is not preventable.

1.1 Overview of Type 1 Diabetes:
  - Type 1 Diabetes results from the immune system mistakenly attacking and destroying insulin-producing beta cells in the pancreas. Without insulin, cells cannot absorb glucose from the bloodstream, leading to elevated blood sugar levels.
  - The exact cause of Type 1 Diabetes is still unknown, but it is believed to involve a combination of genetic predisposition and environmental triggers, such as viral infections or exposure to certain toxins.

1.2 Causes and Symptoms:
  - Genetic factors play a significant role in predisposing individuals to Type 1 Diabetes. Certain genes increase the risk of developing the condition, although not everyone with these genes will develop diabetes.
  - Environmental triggers, such as viral infections or dietary factors, may initiate the autoimmune response that leads to the destruction of beta cells.

- Symptoms of Type 1 Diabetes often develop rapidly and include excessive thirst, frequent urination, sudden weight loss, increased hunger, fatigue, and blurred vision. These symptoms may progress over a few weeks or even days and can be severe enough to prompt medical attention.

1.3 Diagnosis and Initial Steps:
   - Diagnosis of Type 1 Diabetes is typically based on clinical symptoms, blood tests to measure blood glucose levels, and other tests such as glycated hemoglobin (HbA1c) to assess long-term blood sugar control.
   - Upon diagnosis, immediate steps are taken to manage blood sugar levels and prevent complications. Treatment usually involves insulin therapy, which may include multiple daily injections or the use of insulin pumps.
   - Education and support are crucial for individuals and families navigating the challenges of Type 1 Diabetes. Understanding the condition, learning to monitor blood sugar levels, and making dietary and lifestyle adjustments are essential components of managing diabetes effectively.

Understanding the fundamentals of Type 1 Diabetes is the first step towards empowering children and families to take control of their health and navigate the complexities of living with this chronic condition. With proper education, support, and management strategies, individuals with Type 1 Diabetes can lead full and fulfilling lives while effectively managing their health.

Chapter 2

The Importance of Diabetes Management

Managing Type 1 Diabetes effectively is paramount to maintaining good health and preventing long-term complications. This chapter delves into the significance of proactive management, the potential consequences of unmanaged diabetes, and the process of setting goals for effective diabetes care.

2.1 Long-Term Effects of Unmanaged Diabetes:
   Uncontrolled blood sugar levels over time can lead to various complications affecting different organ systems within the body. Chronic hyperglycemia, or high blood sugar, can result in damage to small blood vessels and nerves throughout the body. The consequences of unmanaged diabetes can be severe and may include:

   - Diabetic retinopathy: Damage to the blood vessels in the retina, leading to vision problems and, in severe cases, blindness.
   - Diabetic nephropathy: Kidney damage that can progress to kidney failure, requiring dialysis or kidney transplantation.
   - Diabetic neuropathy: Nerve damage that can cause pain, numbness, tingling, or weakness in the extremities, as well as digestive problems, erectile dysfunction, and other complications.
   - Cardiovascular complications: Diabetes significantly increases the risk of heart disease, stroke, and peripheral

artery disease due to the damaging effects of high blood sugar on the heart and blood vessels.
   - Foot problems: Diabetes can lead to poor circulation and nerve damage in the feet, increasing the risk of foot ulcers, infections, and even amputations if left untreated.

2.2 Benefits of Proactive Management:
   Proactive management of Type 1 Diabetes involves taking proactive steps to control blood sugar levels and prevent complications. This approach can offer numerous benefits, including:

   - Improved quality of life: Proactive diabetes management can help individuals feel better and enjoy a higher quality of life by reducing symptoms such as fatigue, thirst, and frequent urination.
   - Reduced risk of complications: By keeping blood sugar levels within target ranges, individuals can lower their risk of developing diabetes-related complications and improve their long-term health outcomes.
   - Enhanced overall health: Effective diabetes management promotes better overall health by supporting healthy blood pressure, cholesterol levels, and weight management.
   - Greater flexibility and freedom: When diabetes is well-managed, individuals can enjoy more flexibility in their daily activities, dietary choices, and lifestyle decisions.

2.3 Setting Goals for Effective Management:
   Setting realistic and achievable goals is essential for successful diabetes management. Goals should be tailored to individual needs and circumstances, taking into account factors such as age, health status, lifestyle, and personal

preferences. When setting diabetes management goals, consider the following principles:

- Specificity: Goals should be clear, specific, and well-defined, with a clear focus on what needs to be accomplished.
- Measurability: Goals should be measurable so that progress can be tracked and evaluated over time. This may involve monitoring blood sugar levels, tracking dietary habits, or assessing physical activity levels.
- Attainability: Goals should be challenging yet realistic, taking into account individual capabilities, resources, and support systems.
- Relevance: Goals should be relevant to the individual's health priorities, needs, and values, aligning with their overall diabetes management plan.
- Time-bound: Goals should have a defined timeline or deadline for achievement, providing a sense of urgency and accountability.

By setting clear, achievable goals for diabetes management, individuals can empower themselves to take control of their health and work towards better outcomes. Collaborating with healthcare providers, diabetes educators, and support networks can provide valuable guidance and support in setting and achieving these goals effectively.

Chapter 3

Building a Supportive Environment

Navigating Type 1 Diabetes requires more than individual effort—it requires a supportive environment that fosters understanding, encouragement, and collaboration. This chapter explores the crucial role of family support, the importance of educational support in school settings, and the value of community resources and support groups in empowering children with Type 1 Diabetes.

3.1 Family Support and Involvement:
  Family support is the cornerstone of effective diabetes management for children with Type 1 Diabetes. Parents and caregivers play a pivotal role in helping children understand their condition, adhere to treatment regimens, and navigate the daily challenges of living with diabetes. Key aspects of family support include:

  - Education and empowerment: Providing children with age-appropriate information about diabetes empowers them to take an active role in their care. Parents can help children understand the importance of monitoring blood sugar levels, taking insulin, and making healthy lifestyle choices.
  - Emotional support: Living with Type 1 Diabetes can be emotionally challenging for children and families alike. Offering emotional support, empathy, and understanding can help children cope with the stress and anxiety associated with managing a chronic condition.

- Practical assistance: Parents may need to assist younger children with tasks such as blood glucose monitoring, insulin injections, and meal planning. Offering practical assistance and guidance helps children develop the skills they need to manage their diabetes independently as they grow older.

3.2 School Support and Education:

Children with Type 1 Diabetes spend a significant portion of their day at school, making it essential for educators and school staff to understand the condition and provide necessary support. School support for children with Type 1 Diabetes may include:

- Diabetes management plans: Collaborating with healthcare providers and parents to develop individualized diabetes management plans that outline specific care needs, emergency procedures, and accommodations for the classroom and school environment.
- Training and education: Providing training and education to school staff about diabetes management, including recognizing and treating hypoglycemia, administering glucagon in emergencies, and supporting children in monitoring blood sugar levels and administering insulin.
- Advocacy and communication: Advocating for the rights and needs of children with Type 1 Diabetes within the school setting, fostering open communication between parents, educators, and healthcare providers, and addressing any concerns or challenges that may arise.

3.3 Community Resources and Support Groups:
  Community resources and support groups can be invaluable sources of information, encouragement, and connection for families living with Type 1 Diabetes. These resources may include:

  - Diabetes education programs: Local hospitals, clinics, and community organizations may offer diabetes education programs and workshops for children and families, covering topics such as diabetes management, nutrition, and psychosocial support.
  - Support groups: Joining support groups for families affected by Type 1 Diabetes provides opportunities to connect with others facing similar challenges, share experiences, and receive emotional support and practical advice.
  - Advocacy organizations: National and international advocacy organizations dedicated to diabetes awareness and support offer resources, educational materials, and advocacy initiatives aimed at improving diabetes care and quality of life for individuals and families affected by the condition.

By fostering a supportive environment that embraces education, empathy, and collaboration, families, schools, and communities can empower children with Type 1 Diabetes to thrive and achieve their full potential despite the challenges posed by the condition.

Chapter 4

Blood Glucose Monitoring

Blood glucose monitoring is a fundamental aspect of managing Type 1 Diabetes effectively. This chapter delves into the importance of regular monitoring, explores techniques for blood glucose testing, and discusses how to interpret blood glucose results to inform diabetes management decisions.

4.1 Importance of Regular Monitoring:

Regular monitoring of blood glucose levels is essential for individuals with Type 1 Diabetes to understand their body's response to food, physical activity, insulin therapy, and other factors that influence blood sugar levels. Key reasons for regular monitoring include:

- Maintaining target ranges: Monitoring blood glucose levels helps individuals maintain blood sugar levels within target ranges recommended by healthcare providers, reducing the risk of hypo- and hyperglycemia and minimizing the long-term complications associated with diabetes.

- Adjusting treatment regimens: Blood glucose monitoring provides valuable insights into the effectiveness of insulin therapy, dietary choices, and lifestyle habits. By tracking blood sugar levels throughout the day, individuals can make informed adjustments to their treatment regimens to optimize blood sugar control.

- Preventing emergencies: Regular monitoring allows individuals to detect and respond promptly to fluctuations in blood glucose levels, reducing the risk of hypoglycemia (low blood sugar) and hyperglycemia (high blood sugar) emergencies that can lead to serious complications.

4.2 Techniques for Blood Glucose Testing:
   Blood glucose testing can be performed using various methods and devices, depending on individual preferences, lifestyle factors, and treatment goals. Common techniques for blood glucose testing include:

   - Fingerstick blood glucose meters: Portable devices that use a small drop of blood obtained from a fingertip to measure blood glucose levels within seconds. Fingerstick meters are convenient for quick, on-the-go testing and are available in a variety of models with different features.
   - Continuous glucose monitoring (CGM) systems: CGM systems consist of a sensor that is inserted under the skin to measure interstitial glucose levels continuously throughout the day and night. CGM systems provide real-time glucose readings, trend data, and alerts for high and low blood sugar levels, offering valuable insights into blood sugar patterns and trends over time.
   - Flash glucose monitoring systems: Flash glucose monitors use a sensor worn on the skin to measure interstitial glucose levels, which can be scanned with a reader device to obtain glucose readings. Flash glucose monitoring systems offer convenience and discretion, allowing users to access glucose data without the need for routine fingerstick testing.

4.3 Interpreting Blood Glucose Results:
   Interpreting blood glucose results involves understanding the significance of glucose readings in relation to treatment

goals, lifestyle factors, and individual circumstances. Key considerations for interpreting blood glucose results include:

- Target ranges: Healthcare providers establish target ranges for fasting, pre-meal, post-meal, and bedtime blood glucose levels based on individual health status, age, and treatment goals. Blood glucose readings within target ranges indicate good blood sugar control, while readings outside target ranges may require adjustments to treatment regimens.
- Patterns and trends: Monitoring blood glucose levels over time allows individuals to identify patterns and trends in their blood sugar responses to food, physical activity, medication, and other factors. Recognizing patterns can help individuals make informed decisions about insulin dosing, meal timing, and lifestyle modifications to optimize blood sugar control.
- Factors affecting blood glucose: Various factors can influence blood glucose levels, including food choices, carbohydrate intake, physical activity, stress, illness, medications, and hormonal fluctuations. Understanding how these factors affect blood sugar levels enables individuals to anticipate and respond effectively to changes in glucose levels.

By embracing regular blood glucose monitoring as a cornerstone of diabetes management, individuals with Type 1 Diabetes can gain valuable insights into their blood sugar control, make informed decisions about treatment and lifestyle choices, and take proactive steps to optimize their health and well-being.

Chapter 5

Insulin therapy lies at the heart of managing Type 1 Diabetes effectively. This chapter explores the various types of insulin, methods of insulin administration, and the importance of insulin dosage calculation and adjustments in achieving optimal blood sugar control.

5.1 Types of Insulin and Their Action Profiles:
   Insulin is a hormone that helps regulate blood sugar levels by facilitating the uptake of glucose into cells for energy production. Several types of insulin are available, each with unique onset, peak, and duration of action profiles. Common types of insulin include:

  - Rapid-acting insulin: Begins to work within minutes, peaks within 30 minutes to 3 hours, and lasts for 3 to 5 hours. Rapid-acting insulin is typically taken before meals to cover the rise in blood sugar levels after eating.
  - Short-acting (regular) insulin: Begins to work within 30 minutes to 1 hour, peaks within 2 to 4 hours, and lasts for 6 to 8 hours. Short-acting insulin is used to cover meals and may also be administered to correct high blood sugar levels.
  - Intermediate-acting insulin: Begins to work within 1 to 2 hours, peaks within 4 to 12 hours, and lasts for 12 to 18 hours. Intermediate-acting insulin provides basal (background) insulin coverage and helps control blood sugar levels between meals and overnight.

- Long-acting insulin: Begins to work within 1 to 2 hours, has a relatively steady level of activity with no pronounced peak, and lasts for up to 24 hours or longer. Long-acting insulin provides basal insulin coverage and helps maintain stable blood sugar levels throughout the day and night.

5.2 Insulin Administration Methods:
Insulin can be administered via various methods, including syringe and needle, insulin pen, insulin pump, and insulin jet injector. Each method has its advantages and considerations, depending on individual preferences, lifestyle factors, and treatment goals:

- Syringe and needle: Traditional method of insulin administration involving drawing insulin from a vial into a syringe and injecting it into the subcutaneous tissue (fat layer beneath the skin).
- Insulin pen: Prefilled or reusable devices that deliver insulin in precise doses using disposable needles. Insulin pens offer convenience, portability, and ease of use, making them popular choices for many individuals.
- Insulin pump: Small, computerized devices that deliver insulin continuously through a tiny catheter inserted under the skin. Insulin pumps mimic the function of a healthy pancreas by providing basal insulin infusion and allowing for precise mealtime bolus doses.
- Insulin jet injector: Device that uses a high-pressure stream of insulin to penetrate the skin and deliver insulin into the subcutaneous tissue. Insulin jet injectors offer needle-free insulin delivery but may be less commonly used than other methods.

5.3 Insulin Dosage Calculation and Adjustments:
   Determining the appropriate insulin dosage requires careful consideration of various factors, including individual insulin sensitivity, carbohydrate intake, physical activity levels, blood sugar patterns, and treatment goals. Insulin dosage calculation and adjustments involve:

   - Basal insulin: Determining the appropriate basal insulin dose to provide continuous coverage throughout the day and night, adjusting for factors such as fasting blood sugar levels, overnight trends, and basal insulin requirements.
   - Bolus insulin: Calculating mealtime insulin doses (boluses) to cover the carbohydrate content of meals and correct for high blood sugar levels. Bolus insulin doses may be adjusted based on pre-meal blood sugar levels, anticipated carbohydrate intake, and insulin-to-carbohydrate ratios.
   - Correction doses: Administering additional insulin to correct high blood sugar levels, based on correction factors that account for individual insulin sensitivity and target blood sugar levels.

By understanding the principles of insulin therapy, individuals with Type 1 Diabetes can work closely with their healthcare providers to develop personalized insulin regimens that meet their unique needs, lifestyle preferences, and treatment goals. Effective insulin therapy plays a critical role in achieving optimal blood sugar control and promoting overall health and well-being for individuals living with Type 1 Diabetes.

Chapter 6

Nutrition and Meal Planning

Nutrition plays a crucial role in managing Type 1 Diabetes effectively. This chapter explores the principles of balanced nutrition, the role of carbohydrates, proteins, and fats in meal planning, and strategies for managing blood sugar levels through diet.

6.1 Understanding Carbohydrates, Proteins, and Fats:
  - Carbohydrates: Carbohydrates are the primary source of energy for the body and have the most significant impact on blood sugar levels. They are found in foods such as bread, rice, pasta, fruits, vegetables, and dairy products. Individuals with Type 1 Diabetes need to monitor their carbohydrate intake carefully and adjust their insulin doses accordingly to maintain stable blood sugar levels.
  - Proteins: Proteins are essential for building and repairing tissues in the body and can help slow the absorption of carbohydrates, which may help stabilize blood sugar levels. Good sources of protein include lean meats, poultry, fish, eggs, tofu, legumes, and dairy products.
  - Fats: Fats are another source of energy and play a role in hormone production, vitamin absorption, and cell function. While fats do not directly affect blood sugar levels, they can impact overall health and should be consumed in moderation. Healthy fats, such as those found in nuts, seeds, avocados, and olive oil, are preferable to saturated and trans fats found in processed foods and fried foods.

6.2 Meal Planning Strategies for Balanced Nutrition:
  - Carbohydrate counting: Carbohydrate counting involves estimating the amount of carbohydrates in foods and adjusting insulin doses accordingly. This method allows individuals to match their insulin doses to their carbohydrate intake, helping to prevent blood sugar spikes and crashes. Nutrition labels, carbohydrate counting books, and smartphone apps can help individuals track their carbohydrate intake accurately.
  - Glycemic index: The glycemic index (GI) ranks carbohydrate-containing foods based on their effect on blood sugar levels. Foods with a low GI cause a slower, more gradual rise in blood sugar levels, while foods with a high GI cause a rapid spike. Choosing foods with a lower GI can help individuals maintain more stable blood sugar levels throughout the day.
  - Portion control: Controlling portion sizes is essential for managing blood sugar levels and maintaining a healthy weight. Using measuring cups, food scales, and visual cues can help individuals portion out appropriate serving sizes of carbohydrates, proteins, and fats.
  - Meal timing: Consistency in meal timing can help regulate blood sugar levels and insulin requirements. Eating meals and snacks at regular intervals throughout the day can prevent fluctuations in blood sugar levels and reduce the risk of hypoglycemia (low blood sugar) and hyperglycemia (high blood sugar).

6.3 Managing Blood Sugar Levels Through Diet:
  - Balancing carbohydrates: Distributing carbohydrate intake evenly throughout the day can help prevent blood sugar spikes and crashes. Choosing complex

carbohydrates, such as whole grains, fruits, vegetables, and legumes, over refined carbohydrates can also help stabilize blood sugar levels.

- Pairing carbohydrates with protein and fat: Combining carbohydrates with lean protein and healthy fats can help slow the absorption of carbohydrates and prevent rapid spikes in blood sugar levels. Balanced meals and snacks that include a combination of carbohydrates, protein, and fat can help maintain more stable blood sugar levels over time.

- Monitoring post-meal blood sugar levels: Checking blood sugar levels 1-2 hours after meals can help individuals assess the impact of their food choices on blood sugar levels and make adjustments as needed. Keeping a food and blood sugar log can help identify patterns and trends over time, allowing for more informed meal planning and insulin dosing decisions.

By adopting sound nutrition principles and implementing effective meal planning strategies, individuals with Type 1 Diabetes can optimize their blood sugar control, support overall health, and enhance their quality of life. Working with a registered dietitian or certified diabetes educator can provide personalized guidance and support in developing meal plans that meet individual dietary preferences, cultural considerations, and health goals.

Food Item	Serving Size	Carbohydrates (g)	Protein (g)	Fat (g)	Fiber (g)	Glycemic Index
Apple	1 medium (182g)	25	0.5	0.3	4.4	38
Banana	1 medium (118g)	27	1.3	0.4	3.1	51
Orange	1 medium (131g)	15	1.2	0.2	3.1	40
Brown rice	1 cup cooked	45	5	1.6	3.5	50
Quinoa	1 cup cooked	39	8	4	5.2	53
Whole wheat bread	1 slice (28g)	12	2.7	0.9	1.9	69
White bread	1 slice (25g)	12	2.1	0.7	0.8	71
Sweet potato	1 medium (114g)	26	2	0.1	3.9	70
White potato	1 medium (213g)	37	4.3	0.2	4.7	80
Carrots	1 medium (61g)	6	0.3	0.1	1.7	47
Lentils	1 cup cooked	40	18	0.8	15.6	32
Chickpeas	1 cup cooked	45	15	2.4	12.5	33

Food Item	Serving Size	Carbohydrates (g)	Protein (g)	Fat (g)	Fiber (g)	Glycemic Index
Oatmeal (rolled)	1 cup cooked	27	6	3.5	4	55
White rice	1 cup cooked	45	4.2	0.4	0.6	73
Pasta (whole wheat)	1 cup cooked	37	7	1.3	6.3	37
Pasta (white)	1 cup cooked	43	7.5	1.3	2.5	46
Milk (skim)	1 cup (245g)	12	8	0.2	0	32
Greek yogurt (plain)	1 cup (245g)	9	23	0.7	0	11
Almonds	1 ounce (28g)	6	6	14	3.5	-
Broccoli	1 cup chopped (91g)	6	2.6	0.3	2.4	15
Spinach	1 cup raw (30g)	1	0.9	0.1	0.7	0

Glycemic index values may vary depending on factors such as ripeness, cooking method, and food combinations. The values provided in the chart are approximate and can serve as a general guide for meal planning and blood sugar management. Individuals with Type 1 Diabetes should monitor their blood sugar levels and work with healthcare providers to determine the most appropriate foods and meal plans based on their individual needs and preferences.

Chapter 7

Physical Activity and Diabetes

Physical activity plays a vital role in the management of Type 1 Diabetes, contributing to improved blood sugar control, enhanced cardiovascular health, and overall well-being. This chapter explores the benefits of exercise for individuals with Type 1 Diabetes, provides guidelines for safe and effective physical activity, and discusses strategies for balancing insulin, food, and exercise.

7.1 Benefits of Exercise for Diabetes Management:
Engaging in regular physical activity offers numerous benefits for individuals with Type 1 Diabetes, including:
- Improved insulin sensitivity: Exercise helps cells become more responsive to insulin, allowing for better utilization of glucose and improved blood sugar control.
- Lower blood sugar levels: Physical activity can help lower blood sugar levels by increasing glucose uptake into muscles and promoting the release of stored glycogen.
- Weight management: Exercise aids in weight loss and maintenance by burning calories, building lean muscle mass, and increasing metabolism.
- Cardiovascular health: Regular exercise strengthens the heart, lowers blood pressure, improves cholesterol levels, and reduces the risk of heart disease and stroke.
- Stress reduction: Physical activity releases endorphins, neurotransmitters that help alleviate stress, anxiety, and depression, promoting mental well-being.

7.2 Exercise Guidelines and Precautions:

When incorporating exercise into a diabetes management plan, it's essential to consider the following guidelines and precautions:
- Consult with healthcare providers: Before starting a new exercise program, individuals with Type 1 Diabetes should consult with their healthcare team to assess their fitness level, discuss any potential risks or limitations, and develop a personalized exercise plan.
- Choose safe and enjoyable activities: Opt for activities that are safe, enjoyable, and sustainable, such as walking, swimming, cycling, jogging, dancing, or strength training. Be mindful of environmental conditions, such as extreme temperatures or air quality, that may affect exercise safety.
- Monitor blood sugar levels: Check blood sugar levels before, during, and after exercise to prevent hypoglycemia (low blood sugar) and hyperglycemia (high blood sugar). Be prepared to adjust insulin doses, carbohydrate intake, or exercise intensity as needed to maintain stable blood sugar levels.
- Stay hydrated: Drink plenty of water before, during, and after exercise to stay hydrated and prevent dehydration. Avoid sugary sports drinks and opt for water or low-calorie beverages instead.
- Carry emergency supplies: Always carry fast-acting carbohydrates, such as glucose tablets, juice, or candy, to treat hypoglycemia if it occurs during exercise. Wear medical identification jewelry to alert others to your diabetes in case of emergencies.

7.3 Balancing Insulin, Food, and Exercise:
Balancing insulin, food, and exercise is key to achieving optimal blood sugar control before, during, and after

physical activity. Strategies for balancing these factors include:

- Timing insulin doses: Adjust insulin doses based on the timing and intensity of exercise, taking into account factors such as pre-exercise blood sugar levels, anticipated duration and intensity of activity, and insulin action profiles.

- Fueling before exercise: Consume a balanced meal or snack containing carbohydrates, protein, and fat before exercise to provide energy and prevent hypoglycemia. Aim for a carbohydrate-rich snack if blood sugar levels are low before exercise.

- Monitoring during exercise: Monitor blood sugar levels regularly during exercise, especially for prolonged or intense activities. Consider reducing insulin doses or consuming additional carbohydrates if blood sugar levels drop below target ranges.

- Recovery nutrition: Consume a post-exercise snack or meal containing carbohydrates and protein to replenish glycogen stores, repair muscle tissue, and promote recovery. Adjust insulin doses as needed to prevent post-exercise hypoglycemia.

By incorporating regular physical activity into their daily routine and adopting strategies to balance insulin, food, and exercise effectively, individuals with Type 1 Diabetes can enjoy the numerous health benefits of an active lifestyle while maintaining stable blood sugar control and overall well-being. Working closely with healthcare providers and diabetes educators can provide valuable guidance and support in developing safe and personalized exercise plans tailored to individual needs and goals.

Chapter 8

Managing Type 1 Diabetes at school presents unique challenges for children, parents, and educators. This chapter explores the importance of effective communication, collaboration, and education in creating a supportive environment for children with Type 1 Diabetes at school.

8.1 Communicating with School Staff about Diabetes:
   Clear and open communication between parents, healthcare providers, and school staff is essential for ensuring the safety and well-being of children with Type 1 Diabetes while at school. Key aspects of effective communication include:
   - Providing comprehensive information: Parents should communicate important details about their child's diabetes diagnosis, treatment regimen, medication schedule, emergency protocols, and individualized care plan to school administrators, teachers, nurses, coaches, and other relevant staff members.
   - Establishing a communication plan: Establish regular channels of communication between parents and school staff to exchange updates, share concerns, and address any issues related to the child's diabetes management at school. Utilize communication tools such as phone calls, emails, communication logs, and parent-teacher conferences to stay informed and involved.
   - Educating school staff: Offer diabetes education and training sessions for school staff to increase awareness and

understanding of Type 1 Diabetes, its management principles, signs and symptoms of hypo- and hyperglycemia, and appropriate emergency response procedures. Encourage staff members to ask questions, seek clarification, and participate actively in the child's diabetes care plan.

8.2 Creating a Diabetes Management Plan for School:
  A comprehensive diabetes management plan is essential for outlining the child's specific care needs, accommodations, and emergency procedures while at school. Components of a diabetes management plan may include:
  - Medication administration: Specify the child's insulin regimen, dosage instructions, and administration techniques, including the use of insulin pens, pumps, or syringes. Designate trained staff members responsible for administering insulin and monitoring blood sugar levels as needed.
  - Mealtime accommodations: Provide guidance on mealtime routines, carbohydrate counting, snack options, and blood sugar monitoring schedules to ensure consistent blood sugar control throughout the school day. Collaborate with school nutrition services to accommodate dietary restrictions and preferences.
  - Physical activity considerations: Outline strategies for managing blood sugar levels during physical education classes, recess, extracurricular activities, and field trips. Communicate the importance of monitoring blood sugar levels before, during, and after exercise and provide guidelines for preventing and managing hypo- and hyperglycemia during physical activity.

- Emergency protocols: Develop clear protocols for managing diabetes-related emergencies, such as severe hypoglycemia, diabetic ketoacidosis (DKA), or insulin pump failure. Ensure that all school staff members are trained in recognizing emergency signs and symptoms and responding promptly and appropriately to ensure the child's safety and well-being.

8.3 Addressing Challenges and Advocating for Your Child's Needs:

Despite proactive planning and communication, challenges related to managing Type 1 Diabetes at school may arise. Parents and caregivers can take proactive steps to address challenges and advocate for their child's needs by:

- Building partnerships: Foster collaborative relationships with school administrators, teachers, nurses, counselors, and support staff to address concerns, resolve conflicts, and promote a supportive and inclusive school environment for children with Type 1 Diabetes.

- Empowering the child: Educate the child about their diabetes diagnosis, treatment regimen, and self-care responsibilities, empowering them to advocate for their needs, communicate effectively with school staff, and make informed decisions about their health and well-being.

- Seeking support: Seek support from local diabetes organizations, advocacy groups, and parent support networks to connect with other families affected by Type 1 Diabetes, share experiences, access resources, and navigate the challenges of managing diabetes at school.

- Building community: Foster a sense of community and inclusivity by promoting diabetes awareness events, peer support groups, and educational initiatives within the school setting. Encourage collaboration and empathy among students, teachers, and staff members to create a positive and supportive environment where children with Type 1 Diabetes feel accepted, understood, and empowered to succeed academically, socially, and emotionally.

By fostering effective communication, creating a collaborative diabetes management plan, and advocating for their child's needs, parents and caregivers can help ensure a safe, supportive, and inclusive school environment where children with Type 1 Diabetes can thrive academically, socially, and emotionally. Working together with school staff and healthcare providers, families can empower children with Type 1 Diabetes to participate fully in school activities and achieve their full potential despite the challenges posed by their condition.

Empowering the child:

Educate the child about their diabetes diagnosis, treatment regimen, and self-care responsibilities, empowering them to advocate for their needs, communicate effectively with school staff, and make informed decisions about their health and well-being.

Chapter 9

Managing Type 1 Diabetes involves not only physical aspects but also emotional and social challenges that can impact children and their families. This chapter delves into the emotional and social aspects of living with Type 1 Diabetes, offering strategies for coping with the psychological impact, navigating social situations, and building resilience.

9.1 Coping with the Emotional Impact of Diabetes:
   Living with Type 1 Diabetes can evoke a range of emotions, including fear, frustration, anxiety, sadness, and anger. It's essential for children and their families to acknowledge and address these emotions constructively. Strategies for coping with the emotional impact of diabetes include:
   - Open communication: Encourage children to express their feelings and concerns about diabetes openly and honestly with their parents, caregivers, healthcare providers, and peers. Create a supportive and nonjudgmental environment where children feel heard, understood, and validated.
   - Education and empowerment: Provide age-appropriate education about Type 1 Diabetes, its management, and the importance of self-care practices. Empower children to take an active role in managing their diabetes and making informed decisions about their health and well-being.
   - Seeking professional support: Offer access to mental health professionals, counselors, psychologists, or support

groups specializing in pediatric diabetes care. These professionals can provide emotional support, coping strategies, and behavioral interventions to help children and families navigate the challenges of living with diabetes.
   - Stress management techniques: Teach children relaxation techniques, mindfulness practices, deep breathing exercises, or journaling to cope with stress, reduce anxiety, and promote emotional well-being.

9.2 Dealing with Peer Pressure and Stigma:
   Children with Type 1 Diabetes may encounter peer pressure, stigma, and misconceptions about their condition from classmates, friends, and society at large. It's important to address these challenges proactively and promote understanding and acceptance within the community. Strategies for dealing with peer pressure and stigma include:
   - Education and awareness: Educate classmates, teachers, and school staff about Type 1 Diabetes, dispelling myths and misconceptions, and fostering empathy, acceptance, and inclusion. Encourage open dialogue, questions, and discussions to increase awareness and promote a supportive school environment.
   - Advocacy and self-advocacy: Teach children to advocate for themselves and educate others about their diabetes diagnosis, treatment regimen, and individual needs. Encourage assertiveness, self-confidence, and resilience in dealing with peer pressure, teasing, or discriminatory behavior.
   - Building a support network: Encourage children to connect with peers who have Type 1 Diabetes or participate in diabetes camps, support groups, or online

communities where they can share experiences, exchange advice, and find solidarity and encouragement.

- Promoting positive role models: Highlight positive role models and public figures living with Type 1 Diabetes who have overcome challenges, achieved success, and thrived despite their diagnosis. Inspire children to aspire to their dreams and pursue their passions without letting diabetes hold them back.

- Encouraging assertiveness and advocacy: Teach children assertiveness skills and effective communication techniques to assert their needs, correct misconceptions, and advocate for their rights and well-being in social settings.

9.3 Building Resilience and Self-Esteem:
Cultivating resilience and self-esteem is essential for children with Type 1 Diabetes to navigate life's challenges, setbacks, and successes with confidence and optimism. Strategies for building resilience and self-esteem include:

- Emphasizing strengths and achievements: Focus on children's strengths, talents, and accomplishments, celebrating their efforts and progress in managing their diabetes and pursuing their goals. Encourage a growth mindset, resilience, and perseverance in the face of adversity.

- Encouraging independence and autonomy: Support children in taking ownership of their diabetes management and gradually assuming responsibility for self-care tasks, decision-making, and problem-solving. Foster independence, self-reliance, and self-efficacy to empower children to navigate life's challenges with confidence and competence.

- Providing unconditional love and support: Offer unconditional love, acceptance, and support to children with Type 1 Diabetes, emphasizing that their worth and value are not defined by their condition. Create a nurturing and affirming environment where children feel valued, respected, and loved for who they are, beyond their diabetes diagnosis.

- Encouraging self-care practices: Promote self-care activities such as mindfulness, relaxation techniques, and hobbies that empower children to prioritize their emotional well-being and manage stress effectively.

- Celebrating strengths and achievements: Recognize and celebrate children's strengths, talents, and accomplishments in managing their diabetes and overcoming obstacles. Acknowledge their resilience, perseverance, and growth in coping with the demands of their condition.

By addressing the emotional and social aspects of living with Type 1 Diabetes and providing children and families with the tools, resources, and support they need to cope effectively, navigate social challenges, and build resilience, we can help foster a positive and empowering environment where children with Type 1 Diabetes can thrive emotionally, socially, and psychologically, despite the challenges they may face.

Chapter 10

Emergencies and Complications

Managing Type 1 Diabetes involves being prepared to address emergencies and prevent potential complications that may arise. This chapter provides essential information on recognizing, managing, and preventing common diabetes-related emergencies and complications.

10.1 Recognizing and Managing Hypoglycemia:
  Hypoglycemia, or low blood sugar, is a common complication of diabetes that can occur when blood glucose levels drop below normal levels. Symptoms of hypoglycemia include sweating, shakiness, dizziness, confusion, and irritability. Strategies for recognizing and managing hypoglycemia include:
  - Immediate treatment: Instruct individuals with Type 1 Diabetes to consume fast-acting carbohydrates such as glucose tablets, fruit juice, or candy to raise blood sugar levels quickly. Follow up with a snack containing carbohydrates and protein to sustain blood sugar levels.
  - Continuous monitoring: Encourage regular blood glucose monitoring to track changes in blood sugar levels and identify patterns of hypoglycemia. Utilize continuous glucose monitoring (CGM) systems to provide real-time data and alerts for early detection of hypoglycemic episodes.

10.2 Dealing with Hyperglycemia and Diabetic Ketoacidosis (DKA):

Hyperglycemia, or high blood sugar, can lead to diabetic ketoacidosis (DKA), a serious and potentially life-threatening complication of diabetes characterized by high blood ketone levels and metabolic acidosis. Symptoms of DKA include excessive thirst, frequent urination, nausea, vomiting, abdominal pain, and confusion. Strategies for dealing with hyperglycemia and DKA include:

- Fluid and insulin therapy: Administer intravenous fluids and insulin therapy to correct dehydration, lower blood glucose levels, and restore electrolyte balance. Monitor blood ketone levels and acid-base status closely to assess response to treatment and prevent complications.

- Early intervention: Educate individuals with Type 1 Diabetes and their families about the signs and symptoms of hyperglycemia and DKA and the importance of seeking prompt medical attention for early intervention and treatment.

10.3 Preventing and Managing Diabetes-Related Complications:

Long-term complications of Type 1 Diabetes can affect various organs and systems in the body, including the eyes, kidneys, nerves, and cardiovascular system. Strategies for preventing and managing diabetes-related complications include:

- Regular medical check-ups: Schedule regular visits with healthcare providers, including endocrinologists, ophthalmologists, nephrologists, and cardiologists, for comprehensive diabetes care and screening for complications.

- Blood pressure and cholesterol control: Monitor blood pressure and cholesterol levels regularly and implement lifestyle modifications, medications, and interventions to maintain optimal cardiovascular health and reduce the risk of heart disease and stroke.

   - Foot care and neuropathy management: Inspect feet daily for signs of injury, infection, or neuropathy and practice good foot hygiene and care. Seek prompt medical attention for foot ulcers, infections, or other foot problems to prevent complications and promote healing.

By equipping individuals with Type 1 Diabetes and their families with the knowledge, skills, and resources to recognize, manage, and prevent emergencies and complications effectively, we can empower them to take proactive steps to safeguard their health and well-being. Vigilance, education, and early intervention are essential components of comprehensive diabetes care aimed at optimizing outcomes and enhancing quality of life for individuals living with Type 1 Diabetes.

Chapter 11

In the ever-evolving landscape of diabetes management, technology plays a pivotal role in enhancing monitoring, treatment, and overall quality of life for individuals with Type 1 Diabetes. This chapter explores the various technological advancements available to support diabetes management and improve outcomes.

11.1 Continuous Glucose Monitoring (CGM) Systems:
   Continuous Glucose Monitoring (CGM) systems provide real-time monitoring of blood glucose levels, offering valuable insights into trends, patterns, and fluctuations throughout the day and night. Key features and benefits of CGM systems include:
   - Continuous data collection: CGM sensors continuously measure interstitial glucose levels, providing users with up-to-date information on their glucose levels and trends.
   - Alerts and alarms: CGM systems offer customizable alerts and alarms to notify users of impending hypoglycemic or hyperglycemic events, enabling prompt intervention and prevention of severe fluctuations.
   - Trend analysis: CGM data can be analyzed to identify patterns, trends, and correlations between blood glucose levels, meals, physical activity, insulin doses, and other factors, facilitating personalized diabetes management strategies.

11.2 Insulin Pumps and Automated Insulin Delivery Systems:

Insulin pumps and automated insulin delivery systems offer precise and customizable insulin delivery, mimicking the function of the pancreas and optimizing blood glucose control. Key features and benefits of insulin pumps and automated insulin delivery systems include:

- Basal rate delivery: Insulin pumps deliver basal insulin continuously throughout the day to maintain stable blood glucose levels between meals and overnight, providing flexibility and control over insulin dosing.

- Bolus dosing options: Insulin pumps allow users to administer bolus insulin doses to cover meals or correct high blood glucose levels, offering convenience and accuracy in insulin delivery.

- Closed-loop systems: Automated insulin delivery systems, also known as closed-loop systems or hybrid closed-loop systems, combine CGM technology with insulin pump therapy to automate insulin delivery based on real-time glucose data, minimizing the risk of hypo- and hyperglycemia.

11.3 Integration of Technology into Daily Diabetes Care:

Integrating technology into daily diabetes care can streamline management tasks, improve adherence to treatment regimens, and enhance overall quality of life. Strategies for integrating technology into daily diabetes care include:

- Data analysis and interpretation: Utilize diabetes management software and mobile applications to analyze CGM data, track insulin doses, monitor carbohydrate intake, and identify patterns and trends in blood glucose levels over time.

- Remote monitoring and telemedicine: Embrace telemedicine and remote monitoring technologies to facilitate virtual consultations with healthcare providers, diabetes educators, and support teams, enabling timely adjustments to treatment plans and ongoing management support.

   - Education and training: Provide comprehensive education and training on the use of diabetes technology, including CGM systems, insulin pumps, and automated insulin delivery systems, to empower individuals and their families to make informed decisions about their diabetes management.

By leveraging technology to its fullest potential and embracing innovation in diabetes management, individuals with Type 1 Diabetes can achieve improved glycemic control, reduce the risk of acute and long-term complications, and enjoy greater freedom, flexibility, and confidence in managing their diabetes on a daily basis. As technology continues to advance, the future holds promise for further enhancements in diabetes care and empowerment for individuals living with Type 1 Diabetes.

Chapter 12

Transitioning to independence is a significant milestone for adolescents with Type 1 Diabetes as they navigate the complexities of managing their condition while assuming greater responsibility for their health and well-being. This chapter explores the essential aspects of empowering adolescents to transition to independent diabetes management successfully.

12.1 Teaching Self-Care Skills to Adolescents:
Adolescents with Type 1 Diabetes benefit from learning essential self-care skills to manage their condition effectively and promote autonomy in diabetes management. Key self-care skills include:

- Blood glucose monitoring: Educate adolescents on the importance of regular blood glucose monitoring using fingerstick blood glucose meters or continuous glucose monitoring (CGM) systems to track their glucose levels and make informed decisions about insulin dosing and carbohydrate intake.

- Insulin administration: Train adolescents in insulin administration techniques, including insulin pen injection, insulin pump therapy, and dosage calculation, to ensure accurate insulin delivery and optimize glycemic control.

- Carbohydrate counting: Teach adolescents how to count carbohydrates in meals and snacks, estimate portion sizes, and adjust insulin doses accordingly to match their carbohydrate intake and prevent blood glucose fluctuations.

12.2 Gradual Transition to Independent Diabetes Management:

Transitioning to independent diabetes management is a gradual process that requires collaboration between adolescents, parents, healthcare providers, and diabetes educators. Strategies for facilitating a smooth transition include:

- Setting realistic goals: Establish achievable goals and milestones for adolescents to work towards as they transition to independent diabetes management, such as mastering self-care skills, demonstrating competence in insulin dosing, and managing diabetes-related challenges effectively.

- Encouraging self-monitoring: Encourage adolescents to track their blood glucose levels, insulin doses, carbohydrate intake, physical activity, and other relevant factors using diabetes management tools and technology. Review data together to identify trends, patterns, and areas for improvement.

- Providing ongoing support: Offer ongoing guidance, encouragement, and support to adolescents as they navigate the challenges of independent diabetes management. Be available to answer questions, address concerns, and provide reassurance during times of uncertainty or difficulty.

12.3 Supporting Adolescents in Managing Their Diabetes Responsibly:

Empowering adolescents to manage their diabetes responsibly involves fostering a sense of accountability, self-awareness, and resilience. Strategies for supporting adolescents in managing their diabetes responsibly include:

- Encouraging open communication: Create a supportive and nonjudgmental environment where adolescents feel comfortable discussing their diabetes management challenges, concerns, and goals with their parents, healthcare providers, and peers.
- Promoting self-advocacy: Equip adolescents with the knowledge, skills, and confidence to advocate for their diabetes care needs, communicate effectively with healthcare providers, and make informed decisions about their treatment options and lifestyle choices.
- Celebrating achievements: Celebrate adolescents' accomplishments, progress, and efforts in managing their diabetes independently, recognizing their resilience, determination, and growth throughout the transition process.

By empowering adolescents with Type 1 Diabetes to transition to independent diabetes management successfully, we can instill confidence, competence, and resilience in managing their health and well-being as they navigate the journey into adulthood. By fostering a supportive and empowering environment, we can help adolescents thrive and achieve their full potential despite the challenges posed by their condition.

Chapter 13

Living a Full Life with Diabetes

Living with Type 1 Diabetes presents unique challenges, but it also offers opportunities for growth, resilience, and fulfillment. In this chapter, we delve deeper into the strategies and insights that can empower adolescents with Type 1 Diabetes to lead vibrant, meaningful lives while effectively managing their condition.

13.1 Pursuing Hobbies and Interests:
   Engaging in hobbies and interests not only provides enjoyment and fulfillment but also promotes overall well-being and resilience. Adolescents with Type 1 Diabetes can explore a variety of hobbies and interests, such as sports, music, art, writing, cooking, or volunteering, that align with their passions and talents. By pursuing activities they love, adolescents can cultivate a sense of purpose, creativity, and accomplishment, while also fostering connections with others who share similar interests.

   Encouraging adolescents to explore new hobbies and interests expands their horizons, builds confidence, and nurtures a sense of curiosity and exploration. Whether it's learning to play a musical instrument, cultivating a green thumb in the garden, or volunteering for a cause they believe in, adolescents with Type 1 Diabetes can discover new passions and talents that enrich their lives and provide a sense of fulfillment.

13.2 Navigating Social Events and Activities:
   Social events and activities play a vital role in adolescent development and socialization. Adolescents with Type 1 Diabetes can participate in social gatherings, parties, outings, and special occasions with confidence and independence. Strategies for navigating social events include:
   - Planning ahead: Encourage adolescents to plan ahead by checking blood glucose levels, packing diabetes supplies, and anticipating potential challenges or adjustments to their diabetes management routine.
   - Communicating needs: Teach adolescents to communicate their diabetes care needs, dietary preferences, and insulin dosing requirements to friends, family members, and hosts to ensure a safe and inclusive experience.
   - Problem-solving on the go: Equip adolescents with problem-solving skills to address unexpected situations or emergencies that may arise during social events, such as low blood sugar episodes or insulin pump malfunctions.

13.3 Balancing Diabetes Management with Everyday Life:
   Balancing diabetes management with the demands of everyday life requires flexibility, resilience, and self-awareness. Adolescents can integrate diabetes care into their daily routines while pursuing academic, extracurricular, and personal goals. Strategies for balancing diabetes management with everyday life include:
   - Prioritizing self-care: Encourage adolescents to prioritize self-care activities, such as regular blood glucose monitoring, healthy eating, physical activity, and adequate sleep, to maintain optimal health and well-being.

- Seeking support: Foster a supportive network of family, friends, healthcare providers, and peers who understand and respect the challenges of living with Type 1 Diabetes. Encourage adolescents to reach out for support, guidance, and encouragement during times of need or uncertainty.
- Embracing resilience: Cultivate resilience by helping adolescents develop coping skills, problem-solving abilities, and positive coping mechanisms to navigate setbacks, challenges, and transitions with confidence and optimism.

Fostering a growth mindset encourages adolescents to embrace challenges as opportunities for learning and growth, viewing setbacks as temporary obstacles on the path to success. By reframing adversity as a natural part of the human experience, adolescents with Type 1 Diabetes can cultivate resilience, perseverance, and adaptability, empowering them to overcome obstacles.

By embracing a holistic approach to living with Type 1 Diabetes, adolescents can lead fulfilling and meaningful lives characterized by resilience, empowerment, and joy. By nurturing their passions, fostering social connections, and prioritizing self-care, adolescents can thrive and flourish despite the challenges posed by their condition, embracing each day as an opportunity for growth, exploration, and self-discovery.

Chapter 14

Celebrating Successes and MIlestones

Celebrating successes and milestones is an integral part of the journey for adolescents living with Type 1 Diabetes. In this chapter, we explore the importance of recognizing achievements, setting milestones, and fostering a positive outlook on living with diabetes.

14.1 Recognizing Achievements in Diabetes Management:
   Managing Type 1 Diabetes requires dedication, perseverance, and resilience. Adolescents who successfully navigate the challenges of diabetes management deserve recognition and celebration for their achievements, both big and small. Acknowledging accomplishments in diabetes management fosters a sense of pride, motivation, and self-confidence. Celebrate achievements such as:
   - Achieving target blood glucose levels consistently
   - Successfully managing blood sugar fluctuations during physical activity or sports
   - Demonstrating mastery of insulin dosage calculations and adjustments
   - Effectively managing diabetes-related challenges or emergencies

   Celebrating these achievements reinforces positive behaviors, reinforces the importance of consistent diabetes management, and encourages adolescents to continue striving for excellence in their diabetes care.

14.2 Setting and Reaching Milestones:

Setting meaningful milestones empowers adolescents with Type 1 Diabetes to track their progress, set goals, and celebrate their journey towards optimal health and well-being. Milestones can encompass various aspects of diabetes management, personal growth, and lifestyle goals. Encourage adolescents to set and achieve milestones such as:
   - Graduating to a higher level of diabetes management independence
   - Successfully navigating a social event or outing while managing diabetes effectively
   - Incorporating new healthy habits into their daily routine, such as regular exercise or mindful eating
   - Completing diabetes education programs or certifications

   Reaching milestones provides a sense of accomplishment, reinforces positive behaviors, and builds momentum for continued progress and growth in diabetes management and overall well-being.

14.3 Fostering a Positive Outlook on Living with Diabetes:
   Cultivating a positive outlook on living with Type 1 Diabetes is essential for adolescents to thrive emotionally, mentally, and socially. Encourage adolescents to embrace their diabetes journey with optimism, resilience, and gratitude. Strategies for fostering a positive outlook include:
   - Practicing self-compassion and acceptance: Encourage adolescents to embrace self-compassion and accept diabetes as part of their identity without judgment or self-criticism. Emphasize the importance of treating themselves

with kindness, patience, and understanding, especially during challenging times.

- Finding joy and gratitude in daily life: Encourage adolescents to focus on the positive aspects of their diabetes journey, such as the supportive relationships they've built, the lessons they've learned, and the personal growth they've experienced. Encourage them to cultivate gratitude for the blessings and opportunities in their lives, despite the challenges they may face.

- Engaging in activities that bring joy and fulfillment: Encourage adolescents to prioritize activities that bring them joy, fulfillment, and a sense of purpose, whether it's spending time with loved ones, pursuing hobbies and interests, or giving back to their community.

By fostering a positive outlook on living with diabetes, adolescents can develop resilience, adaptability, and a sense of empowerment in navigating life's challenges. They can embrace their diabetes journey with courage and optimism, recognizing that they are capable of overcoming obstacles and achieving their dreams, one milestone at a time.

Celebrating successes and milestones empowers adolescents with Type 1 Diabetes to embrace their journey with optimism, resilience, and gratitude. By recognizing achievements, setting meaningful milestones, and fostering a positive outlook, adolescents can thrive emotionally, mentally, and socially, living life to the fullest despite the challenges posed by their condition.

Chapter 15

Looking Towards the Future

As adolescents with Type 1 Diabetes transition into adulthood, they embark on a journey filled with hope, opportunities, and advancements in diabetes care. In this chapter, we explore the evolving landscape of diabetes research, treatment options, and empowering strategies for adolescents to embrace the future with confidence and optimism.

15.1 Advances in Diabetes Research and Treatment:
  The field of diabetes research continues to evolve, offering promising advancements in treatment modalities, technology, and understanding of the underlying mechanisms of Type 1 Diabetes. Adolescents with Type 1 Diabetes can look towards the future with optimism, knowing that ongoing research holds the potential for:
  - Improved insulin delivery systems: Advances in insulin pump technology, automated insulin delivery systems, and closed-loop systems offer greater precision, flexibility, and convenience in insulin administration, enhancing glycemic control and quality of life.
  - Novel therapies and interventions: Researchers are exploring innovative therapies and interventions, such as beta cell transplantation, immunotherapy, and gene editing techniques, aimed at preserving beta cell function, halting autoimmune destruction, and achieving diabetes remission.
  - Personalized medicine approaches: Tailored treatment approaches based on individual genetic, metabolic, and lifestyle factors hold promise for optimizing diabetes

management, minimizing complications, and enhancing outcomes for adolescents with Type 1 Diabetes.

By staying informed about the latest developments in diabetes research and treatment, adolescents can make informed decisions about their diabetes care and remain hopeful for future advancements that may transform the landscape of diabetes management.

15.2 Hope for a Cure:
While Type 1 Diabetes is currently a chronic condition without a cure, ongoing research efforts worldwide are dedicated to finding a cure and eradicating the disease. Adolescents with Type 1 Diabetes can hold onto hope for a cure, knowing that dedicated researchers and organizations are working tirelessly towards this common goal. Strategies for fostering hope for a cure include:
- Participating in clinical trials and research studies: Adolescents can contribute to diabetes research by participating in clinical trials, research studies, and advocacy efforts aimed at advancing scientific understanding and treatment options for Type 1 Diabetes.
- Supporting diabetes advocacy and awareness initiatives: Engaging in diabetes advocacy and awareness initiatives empowers adolescents to raise awareness, promote research funding, and advocate for policies that support diabetes research, education, and access to care.
- Connecting with the diabetes community: Building connections with other individuals and families affected by Type 1 Diabetes provides a sense of solidarity, support, and shared purpose in the quest for a cure. Participating in community events, support groups, and online forums fosters a sense of belonging and hope for the future.

By actively engaging in diabetes advocacy, research participation, and community involvement, adolescents can contribute to the collective efforts towards finding a cure for Type 1 Diabetes and inspiring hope for a future free from the burdens of the disease.

15.3 Empowering Adolescents to Thrive:
As adolescents with Type 1 Diabetes look towards the future, they can embrace a mindset of empowerment, resilience, and self-advocacy. Empowering strategies for adolescents to thrive include:
- Taking ownership of their health: Encourage adolescents to take an active role in managing their diabetes, advocating for their healthcare needs, and making informed decisions about their treatment options and lifestyle choices.
- Setting goals and pursuing dreams: Support adolescents in setting meaningful goals, pursuing their passions, and envisioning a future filled with possibilities and opportunities for personal and professional growth.
- Building a support network: Foster connections with healthcare providers, diabetes educators, mentors, and peers who understand and support their journey with Type 1 Diabetes. Surrounding themselves with a supportive network provides encouragement, guidance, and reassurance along the way.

By embracing a future-oriented mindset, adolescents with Type 1 Diabetes can navigate life's challenges with resilience, optimism, and determination, knowing that they have the knowledge, skills, and support to thrive despite the challenges posed by their condition.

As adolescents with Type 1 Diabetes embark on their journey towards adulthood, they can look towards the future with hope, optimism, and empowerment. By staying informed about advances in diabetes research and treatment, fostering hope for a cure, and embracing strategies for personal growth and resilience, adolescents can navigate the uncertainties of the future with confidence, knowing that they are equipped to face whatever challenges may come their way.

15.4 Cultivating Resilience:
Despite the challenges on the path towards a cure for Type 1 Diabetes, adolescents can find strength in their resilience. Building resilience involves developing inner fortitude, coping mechanisms, and a positive outlook that enables adolescents to confront life's trials with perseverance and adaptability. By reframing setbacks as opportunities for growth and learning, adolescents can navigate hurdles with resilience and emerge stronger and more resilient than before.

15.5 Inspiring Change:
Adolescents with Type 1 Diabetes hold the potential to inspire others and effect positive change in the diabetes community and beyond. Through storytelling, advocacy, and support for fellow individuals living with diabetes, adolescents can amplify their voices and drive impactful transformations. By leading by example and embodying qualities of resilience, empowerment, and advocacy, adolescents can inspire hope, foster connections, and leave a lasting legacy of courage and compassion for generations to come.

Glossary of Terms

1. Type 1 Diabetes: A chronic autoimmune condition in which the pancreas produces little to no insulin, requiring lifelong insulin therapy for blood sugar control.

2. Insulin: A hormone produced by the pancreas that regulates blood sugar levels by facilitating the uptake of glucose into cells for energy or storage.

3. Blood Glucose: The concentration of glucose (sugar) present in the bloodstream, measured in milligrams per deciliter (mg/dL) or millimoles per liter (mmol/L).

4. Hypoglycemia: A condition characterized by low blood glucose levels (typically below 70 mg/dL), resulting in symptoms such as shakiness, sweating, confusion, and fatigue.

5. Hyperglycemia: A condition characterized by high blood glucose levels, often exceeding normal ranges (typically above 180 mg/dL), resulting in symptoms such as increased thirst, frequent urination, and blurred vision.

6. Carbohydrates: The main macronutrient found in food, including sugars, starches, and fiber, which are broken down into glucose during digestion and impact blood sugar levels.

7. Insulin Therapy: The primary treatment for Type 1 Diabetes, involving the administration of insulin via

injections, insulin pumps, or inhalation to regulate blood sugar levels.

8. Continuous Glucose Monitoring (CGM): A system that continuously monitors blood glucose levels throughout the day and night, providing real-time data and trend information to aid in diabetes management.

9. Insulin Pump: A small electronic device worn externally that delivers insulin continuously through a catheter placed under the skin, offering precise insulin dosing and flexibility in insulin delivery.

10. A1C Test: A blood test that measures average blood glucose levels over the past two to three months, providing an indicator of long-term blood sugar control.

11. Diabetes Management Plan: A personalized plan developed in collaboration with healthcare providers to guide diabetes care, including blood glucose monitoring, insulin dosing, meal planning, physical activity, and emergency protocols.

12. Ketones: Byproducts of the breakdown of fatty acids when insulin levels are insufficient, potentially leading to diabetic ketoacidosis (DKA), a serious complication of untreated or poorly managed Type 1 Diabetes.

13. Hemoglobin: A protein in red blood cells that binds to glucose, providing a measure of average blood glucose levels over time in the A1C test.

Sample Meal Plans

Sample Meal Plan 1:

Breakfast:
- Scrambled eggs with spinach and tomatoes
- Whole grain toast with avocado spread
- Sliced strawberries
- Water or unsweetened almond milk

Mid-Morning Snack:
- Apple slices with peanut butter

Lunch:
- Turkey and cheese whole grain wrap with lettuce and cucumber
- Baby carrots with hummus
- Greek yogurt with mixed berries
- Water or herbal tea

Afternoon Snack:
- Celery sticks with cream cheese

Dinner:
- Grilled chicken breast with roasted sweet potatoes and broccoli
- Quinoa salad with bell peppers, cucumbers, and vinaigrette dressing
- Water or sparkling water with lemon

Evening Snack:
- Cottage cheese with pineapple chunks

Sample Meal Plan 2:

Breakfast:
- Oatmeal topped with sliced bananas and walnuts
- Hard-boiled egg
- Orange slices
- Water or low-fat milk

Mid-Morning Snack:
- Whole grain crackers with cheese slices

Lunch:
- Spinach and strawberry salad with grilled chicken, almonds, and balsamic vinaigrette
- Whole grain roll
- Carrot sticks with hummus
- Water or unsweetened iced tea

Afternoon Snack:
- Rice cakes with almond butter

Dinner:
- Baked salmon with quinoa pilaf and steamed green beans
- Mixed green salad with cherry tomatoes and avocado
- Water or sparkling water with lime

Evening Snack:
- Greek yogurt with sliced peaches

Sample Meal Plan 3:

Breakfast:
- Whole grain pancakes with blueberries and maple syrup
- Scrambled tofu with spinach and mushrooms
- Water or unsweetened coconut water

Mid-Morning Snack:
- Cottage cheese with pineapple chunks

Lunch:
- Black bean and vegetable burrito bowl with brown rice, salsa, avocado, and lettuce
- Corn tortilla chips with guacamole
- Water or herbal tea

Afternoon Snack:
- Edamame beans with sea salt

Dinner:
- Turkey meatballs with whole wheat spaghetti and marinara sauce
- Steamed broccoli florets
- Water or unsweetened iced tea

Evening Snack:
- Frozen grapes

Consulting with a registered dietitian or healthcare provider can help customize meal plans to meet the specific dietary and nutritional requirements of children with Type 1 Diabetes.

Blood Glucose Log

Date	Time	Blood Glucose (mg/dl)	Insulin Dose (mg/dl)	Carb Intake (g)	Physical Activity	Notes

Emergency Action Plan for

---

with Type 1 Diabetes

Emergency Contacts:

1. Parent/Guardian:
2. Healthcare Provider:
3. Emergency Services: 911

Medical Information:

- Child's Name:
- Date of Birth:
- Diagnosis: Type 1 Diabetes
- Medications: Insulin, Glucagon
- Allergies:

Emergency Procedures:

1. Hypoglycemia (Low Blood Sugar):
  - Signs and Symptoms: Shakiness, sweating, confusion, irritability, dizziness, hunger, weakness.
   - Treatment:
    - Administer fast-acting carbohydrates: juice, glucose gel, or glucose tablets.
    - Recheck blood glucose levels after 15 minutes. If still low, repeat treatment.

- If unconscious or unable to swallow, administer glucagon injection and call emergency services.
   - Follow-up: Offer a snack with protein and carbohydrates to prevent rebound hypoglycemia.

2. Hyperglycemia (High Blood Sugar):
  - Signs and Symptoms: Increased thirst, frequent urination, blurred vision, fatigue, nausea, vomiting.
   - Treatment:
    - Check blood glucose levels.
    - Administer insulin as prescribed by healthcare provider.
    - Encourage fluid intake, preferably water.
    - Monitor ketone levels if indicated.
    - Seek medical attention if blood glucose levels remain high or if ketones are present.

3. Severe Hypoglycemia/Unconsciousness:
  - Signs and Symptoms: Loss of consciousness, seizures, inability to swallow.
   - Treatment:
    - Administer glucagon injection as directed by healthcare provider.
    - Call emergency services immediately.
    - Do not attempt to force feed or administer anything by mouth if the child is unconscious.

4. Severe Hyperglycemia/Ketoacidosis:
  - Signs and Symptoms: Excessive thirst, fruity breath odor, rapid breathing, confusion, abdominal pain.
   - Treatment:
    - Administer insulin as directed by healthcare provider.
    - Encourage fluid intake, preferably water.
    - Monitor blood glucose and ketone levels.

   - Seek immediate medical attention if symptoms persist or worsen.

Additional Instructions:
- Keep emergency supplies readily accessible at all times, including fast-acting carbohydrates, glucagon emergency kit, blood glucose meter, insulin, and ketone testing supplies.
- Educate family members, caregivers, and school personnel about the signs, symptoms, and treatment of hypo- and hyperglycemia.
- Update the emergency action plan regularly based on changes in the child's condition or treatment plan.

Review and Practice:
Review and practice emergency procedures regularly with family members, caregivers, and school personnel to ensure readiness in case of an emergency.

This emergency action plan should be customized based on the child's specific medical history, treatment regimen, and healthcare provider's recommendations. It's essential to keep a printed copy of the emergency action plan in easily accessible locations, such as at home, school, and when traveling, to ensure quick and appropriate response during emergencies related to Type 1 Diabetes.

School Diabetes Management Plan for

____

Student Information:
- Student's Name:
- Date of Birth:
- Grade/Class:
- School:
- Parent/Guardian:
- Emergency Contact:
- Healthcare Provider:

Diabetes Information:
- Type of Diabetes: Type 1 Diabetes
- Date of Diagnosis:
- Treatment Plan: Insulin therapy, blood glucose monitoring, carbohydrate counting, etc.
- Emergency Care Plan: Include instructions for hypo- and hyperglycemia management and severe episodes.

Daily Management:
1. Blood Glucose Monitoring:
   - Frequency:
   - Location:
   - Equipment:

2. Insulin Administration:
   - Dosage:
   - Injection Sites:
   - Storage:

3. Meal and Snack Management:
   - Meal Planning:
   - Snack Times:

4. Physical Activity:
   - Guidelines:
   - Emergency Supplies:

Emergency Procedures:
- Hypoglycemia (Low Blood Sugar):
- Hyperglycemia (High Blood Sugar):
- Severe Episodes:

Communication Plan:
- Parent/School Communication:
- Emergency Contacts:

Training and Education:
- Staff Training:
- Student Education:

Field Trips and Extracurricular Activities:
- Guidelines:

Regularly review and update the school diabetes management plan in collaboration with parents/guardians, healthcare providers, and school personnel to address any changes in the child's condition or treatment regimen.

FAQ and Common Concerns

1. What is Type 1 Diabetes, and how is it different from Type 2 Diabetes?
   - Type 1 Diabetes is an autoimmune condition where the body's immune system attacks insulin-producing cells in the pancreas. It requires insulin therapy for blood sugar control. Type 2 Diabetes, on the other hand, is characterized by insulin resistance and can often be managed with lifestyle changes and medications.

2. How is Type 1 Diabetes diagnosed in children?
   - Type 1 Diabetes is typically diagnosed through blood tests that measure blood glucose levels and detect the presence of autoantibodies associated with pancreatic beta-cell destruction.

3. What are the symptoms of Type 1 Diabetes in children?
   - Common symptoms include excessive thirst, frequent urination, unexplained weight loss, fatigue, irritability, and blurred vision. Children may also experience increased hunger, sudden mood changes, and recurrent infections.

4. How is blood glucose monitored in children with Type 1 Diabetes?
   - Blood glucose levels are monitored using a blood glucose meter, which requires a small blood sample obtained through finger pricks. Continuous glucose monitoring (CGM) systems can also be used to track blood glucose levels continuously throughout the day and night.

5. What role does insulin play in managing Type 1 Diabetes?
   - Insulin is essential for regulating blood sugar levels by facilitating the uptake of glucose into cells for energy. Children with Type 1 Diabetes require insulin therapy to replace the insulin their bodies cannot produce.

6. How do children with Type 1 Diabetes manage their diet?
   - Children with Type 1 Diabetes often follow a balanced meal plan that includes a variety of foods while considering carbohydrate intake for blood sugar control. They may use carbohydrate counting or the glycemic index to help manage their diet effectively.

7. What are the risks associated with uncontrolled blood sugar levels in children with Type 1 Diabetes?
   - Uncontrolled blood sugar levels can lead to short-term complications such as hypoglycemia (low blood sugar) and hyperglycemia (high blood sugar), as well as long-term complications including cardiovascular disease, kidney damage, nerve damage, and eye problems.

8. How can parents and caregivers support children with Type 1 Diabetes at school?
   - Parents and caregivers can work with school staff to develop a comprehensive diabetes management plan that includes blood glucose monitoring, insulin administration, meal planning, and emergency procedures. Educating teachers and school personnel about the child's needs and ensuring access to necessary supplies and accommodations are also essential.

9. What should parents do in case of an emergency related to Type 1 Diabetes?
   - Parents should have a written emergency action plan in place outlining procedures for managing hypo- and hyperglycemia, administering glucagon if necessary, and seeking medical assistance promptly. It's crucial to educate family members, caregivers, and school personnel about the child's emergency protocols.

10. Are there any advancements in Type 1 Diabetes treatment and management?
   - Yes, ongoing research has led to advancements in insulin delivery methods, continuous glucose monitoring technology, and potential immunotherapies aimed at preserving pancreatic function and improving blood sugar control. It's important for families to stay informed about new developments and discuss treatment options with healthcare providers.

Technology Resources

1. Continuous Glucose Monitoring (CGM) Systems:
   - CGM systems continuously monitor blood glucose levels throughout the day and night, providing real-time data and trends. Examples include Dexcom G6, Medtronic Guardian Connect, and Freestyle Libre.

2. Insulin Pumps:
   - Insulin pumps deliver insulin continuously throughout the day, offering flexibility in insulin dosing and mealtime boluses. They can be programmed to deliver basal rates and boluses based on individual insulin needs. Some popular insulin pumps include Medtronic MiniMed 670G, Tandem t:slim X2, and Omnipod.

3. Mobile Apps:
   - There are various mobile apps available for diabetes management, including apps for tracking blood glucose levels, carbohydrate intake, insulin doses, and physical activity. Some apps also offer features such as data visualization, trend analysis, and integration with CGM systems. Examples include mySugr, Glucose Buddy, and Sugarmate.

4. Telemedicine Platforms:
   - Telemedicine platforms allow individuals with Type 1 Diabetes to connect with healthcare providers remotely for consultations, monitoring, and education. These platforms can be particularly helpful for accessing specialized care and support from endocrinologists and diabetes educators.

5. Educational Websites and Online Communities:
   - Websites and online communities dedicated to diabetes education and support offer valuable resources, articles, webinars, and forums where individuals and families can learn about diabetes management, share experiences, and connect with others facing similar challenges. Examples include Beyond Type 1, Diabetes Daily, and Children with Diabetes.

6. Artificial Pancreas Systems:
   - Artificial pancreas systems, also known as closed-loop systems, automate insulin delivery based on real-time glucose monitoring data, aiming to mimic the function of a healthy pancreas. These systems can help improve blood glucose control and reduce the risk of hypoglycemia. Examples include the Tandem Control-IQ and Medtronic MiniMed 780G.

7. Wearable Technology:
   - Wearable devices, such as smartwatches and fitness trackers, can be integrated with diabetes management apps and CGM systems, allowing users to monitor blood glucose levels, receive alerts and notifications, and track physical activity and sleep patterns conveniently.

8. Online Educational Courses and Webinars:
   - Many organizations offer online educational courses and webinars on various aspects of diabetes management, including nutrition, insulin therapy, exercise, and coping strategies. These resources can help individuals and families enhance their diabetes knowledge and skills from the comfort of their homes.

Insurance and Financial Assistance

1. Health Insurance Navigation:
   - Healthcare.gov: The official health insurance marketplace offers information about health insurance options, coverage, and enrollment assistance.
   - Local Health Insurance Assistance Programs: Many states offer assistance programs and resources to help individuals and families navigate health insurance options and enroll in coverage.

2. Prescription Assistance Programs:
   - Partnership for Prescription Assistance (PPA): PPA provides access to prescription assistance programs offered by pharmaceutical companies, offering discounted or free medications, including insulin and diabetes supplies.
   - RxAssist: RxAssist offers information about patient assistance programs and resources to help individuals access affordable prescription medications.

3. Government Assistance Programs:
   - Medicaid: Medicaid provides health coverage to eligible low-income individuals and families, including children with Type 1 Diabetes. Eligibility requirements vary by state.
   - Children's Health Insurance Program (CHIP): CHIP offers low-cost health coverage for children in families that do not qualify for Medicaid but cannot afford private insurance.

4. Nonprofit Organizations:
   - JDRF (Juvenile Diabetes Research Foundation): JDRF offers resources and support for individuals and families affected by Type 1 Diabetes, including advocacy efforts, educational programs, and fundraising events.
   - American Diabetes Association (ADA): ADA provides information and resources on diabetes management, advocacy, and support services for individuals and families living with diabetes.

5. Financial Assistance Programs:
   - Patient Advocate Foundation (PAF): PAF offers financial assistance programs and resources to help patients access healthcare services, including assistance with insurance premiums, copayments, and medical debt.
   - Diabetes Foundation: Some local and national diabetes foundations offer financial assistance programs and grants to help individuals and families cover the costs of diabetes care and supplies.

6. Pharmaceutical Assistance Programs:
   - Insulin Manufacturer Assistance Programs: Pharmaceutical companies that manufacture insulin may offer patient assistance programs to help individuals access insulin at reduced or no cost. Contact the manufacturer directly for information about available programs and eligibility criteria.

7. Community Health Centers:
   - Federally Qualified Health Centers (FQHCs): FQHCs
provide comprehensive healthcare services, including
primary care, dental care, and behavioral health services, to
underserved populations, regardless of insurance status or
ability to pay.

8. Local Social Services Agencies:
   - Local social services agencies may offer assistance
programs and resources to help individuals and families
access healthcare services, prescription medications, and
other essential needs. Contact your local social services
department for information about available programs and
eligibility requirements.

Epilogue

As we conclude this journey through the complexities of managing Type 1 Diabetes in children, it's essential to reflect on the progress made and the challenges that lie ahead. We've explored the intricacies of blood glucose monitoring, insulin therapy, nutrition management, and the emotional and social aspects of living with diabetes. Through it all, we've witnessed the resilience and determination of children and families facing this chronic condition head-on.

In the time since we embarked on this exploration, advancements in technology have revolutionized diabetes management, offering innovative tools and therapies to improve blood sugar control and enhance quality of life. Continuous glucose monitoring systems, insulin pumps, and artificial pancreas systems have become integral parts of diabetes care, providing real-time data and personalized treatment options.

Moreover, the diabetes community has grown stronger, with advocacy efforts driving awareness, research, and support for individuals and families affected by Type 1 Diabetes. Through education, empowerment, and collaboration, we continue to strive for better outcomes and a brighter future for those living with diabetes.

As we look ahead, it's important to remember that the journey doesn't end here. There will be triumphs and setbacks, moments of joy and moments of frustration. But with knowledge, support, and perseverance, we can face the challenges of Type 1 Diabetes with courage and determination.

To all those who have shared in this journey, whether as caregivers, healthcare providers, researchers, or individuals living with diabetes, your dedication and strength inspire us all. Together, we stand united in our pursuit of better treatments, improved outcomes, and ultimately, a cure for Type 1 Diabetes.

As the pages of this book come to a close, let us carry forward the lessons learned, the connections made, and the hope that fuels our resolve. For in the face of adversity, it is our collective resilience and determination that will guide us toward a future where diabetes no longer casts its shadow.

May this journey be a testament to the power of community, the spirit of resilience, and the unwavering hope that sustains us all.

With gratitude and optimism,

Alexander Wellington

About the Author

Alexander Wellington is a passionate advocate for health and wellness, with a particular focus on diabetes education and advocacy. Alexander is committed to empowering individuals and families affected by Type 1 Diabetes.

Throughout the years, Alexander has tried to bridge the gap between medical knowledge and practical application, providing valuable insights and resources to help individuals and families navigate the complexities of diabetes care. He is a firm believer in the power of education, advocacy, and community support in improving outcomes and quality of life for those living with diabetes.

As an author, Alexander is dedicated to sharing his insights to empower readers with the knowledge and tools they need to thrive in their diabetes journey. Through his writing, he seeks to inspire hope, foster resilience, and advocate for positive change in diabetes care and management.